<u>Foreword</u>

School teaches you a wealth of information, and that knowledge-base is extremely important. But, equally important are the real-life situations you will be exposed to - one's that are not commonly taught in school. It's one thing to read about torn PCLs or disc herniations, but it's a whole new world when you have a patient with a ton of questions about it. Furthermore, private practice also opens up a whole new world in terms of actually running a business – becoming proficient in dealing with insurance, billing, scheduling, taxes, accounting, etc. We created this book to help prepare you for these situations. These are real patients that I saw, with real questions and conditions that walked in the first year of being open. There are concepts, such as relationship-building, patient-focused care, and empathy that were touched upon in school, but made much more apparent in private practice. This book also includes business-related reflections related to starting and running a new business. I want to share what we learned so far in the hopes that you will be able to utilize anything we learned for your greater good.

1

Introduction

The following is a compilation of information on the first year of being in private practice. My business partner Drew Accomando and I opened our chiropractic / fitness clinic on March 20th, 2017. It was on that day that I began the process. I recorded what questions the first 100 patients asked me and what medical conditions they had in the past or when I saw them. The goal was to create something to help expose future chiropractors, physicians, or other manual therapists to real world scenarios. This information can offer great insight on what to expect, such as what questions might be asked and what conditions might walk in. It's not always what you learn in school that's important, but how effectively you can apply and communicate it. This can help you prepare for the unexpected. One can look at the lists and see how they would have answered the questions or what they would do for various conditions.

I also wrote down a list of things we didn't expect (or just didn't know a lot about) throughout the process of starting and running our own business and created a list of recommendations. This can help further prepare future practitioners and enable them to be as confident and ready as possible, whether it be as a new doc in general or as one opening a new practice. As you'll soon see, the questions and conditions were highly varied.

To understand why some questions were asked, it's important to first highlight how Drew and I run our facility and the treatment modalities we tend to use. We offer personal training and chiropractic services. I do a lot of soft tissue work (cupping, instrument-assisted soft tissue mobilization, pin-and-stretch), Flexion-and-Distraction, nutritional counseling, adjustments, acupuncture, dry needling, and rehabilitation. I'll occasionally use E-stim, ice/heat, activator, and kinesio-taping. Drew oversees all the personal training (weight loss, injury prevention, sports performance, nutritional counseling) and performs a good deal of the rehabilitation. Now, here we go!

2

Questions

These are the questions that the first 100 patients asked me:

Knots:

1. What is a knot?
2. Can knots cause radiation?
3. Can knots go away?
4. How do knots form?
5. Were you able to see knots on cadaver dissections?
6. Are knots present in the same place on everybody?
7. Why are knots so tender?

Fascia:

1. What is fascia?
2. Can you give me an analogy for fascia?
3. Is fascia only located in the foot?
4. What is fascia made of?
5. What does fascia do?
6. Is it my fascia that hurts or my muscles?

Food, Supplements, or Diets:

1. Is supplementing with ALA (Alpha Lipoic Acid) good?
2. Do you know anything about molasses?
3. What are some natural supplements to improve my sleep?
4. What do you think about ketone sticks?
5. What kind of probiotics do you recommend?
6. What do you think will help me lose weight faster, the ketogenic diet or the paleo diet?
7. Does coffee dehydrate you?
8. Would you recommend that I continue the ketogenic diet?
9. How do you feel about growth hormone supplementation?
10. Does drinking Branched-Chain Amino Acids count as breaking a fast?
11. What exactly is cholesterol and why is it bad for you?
12. How do you feel about dairy?
13. How often should I eat?
14. How do you feel about HMB (Hydroxy-Methyl-Butyrate) supplementation?
15. If you would recommend 3 supplements what would they be?
16. Are you familiar with the blood type diet?
17. Why do I feel the tingling in my face after taking beta-alanine?

18. *Patient preparing for a half-marathon* What do you think is the best energy bar for me to take during the run and just before the run?
19. Should I eat more carbs or more fat throughout the day?
20. Can you give B12 shots?
21. Have you ever heard of the low salicylic acid diet?
22. When should I have a protein shake?
23. What's the benefit of supplementing with fish oil?
24. If I get plenty of sun exposure, would I need to supplement with Vitamin D?
25. What supplements do you take?
26. Why did you choose to work with this supplement company (Jarrow)?

Chiropractic, Adjustments, Alignments, etc.

1. What is an adjustment / How does an adjustment work? **(The most popular question of all)**
2. Can chiropractic help with ear infections?
3. Can adjustments make you sleep better?
4. Are my neck and back pain related?
5. What is an inversion table used for?
6. Can my hips be misaligned?

7. Are there good popping sounds and bad popping sounds?
8. Why is rotation the worst way to adjust the neck?
9. Does cracking lead to arthritis?
10. Do you adjust everybody?
11. Is self-adjusting bad?
12. What exactly are you feeling [palpating] for?
13. What causes that cracking sound?
14. Can adjustments cause a disc herniation?
15. Is an activator more or less effective than an adjustment?
16. Can my IT-Band be causing my knee pain?
17. Why do I stand with my knees hyperextended?
18. Is it better to get adjusted before or after a workout?
19. Can you read my MRI results (also got questions for CT, X-ray, ultrasound)?
20. Should I get imaged (X-ray, MRI, etc) right away?
21. Can my hamstrings be causing my sciatica?
22. Is there anything I can do to improve my posture?
23. Can you prescribe medications?
24. Can you write me a script for a stand-up table?
25. Can you prescribe marijuana?
26. Are chiropractors trained in yoga?

27. What are some stretches for the piriformis?
28. How much schooling did you have to go through?
29. How long does it take for an adjustment to work?
30. Do you need a script before you start treating me?
31. What's the difference between you and a physical therapist?
32. Did you guys (chiropractors) have to go through residency?

Medical Conditions

1. What exactly is a microdiscectomy?
2. How do I know if my pain is from sciatica or not?
3. *Patient with large scar on triceps muscle*- Why does the muscle twitch sometimes?
4. Is my forearm tightness causing my hand numbness/tingling?
5. How can my hand numbness come from my neck pain?
6. Is sciatica real?
7. What do they do for a coccyx fracture?
8. What's a good treatment for bunions?
9. Why does the radiation down my legs switch sides?
10. *Patient with plantar fasciitis* What can I do to help this on my own?

11. *Patient with cervical spine strain* How long will my neck pain last?
12. What exactly is a strain, an over-stretch or an over-contraction?
13. How long does acute disc pain usually last?
14. Can my period cause knee swelling?
15. What would it mean if my reflexes weren't there?
16. What's a spinal concussion?
17. Can osteoporosis be localized?
18. How do you know if it's an "itis" or an "osis"?
19. Can my shoes be aggravating my knee pain?
20. Can my radiculopathy be causing me to get sore faster?
21. What exactly is stenosis?
22. Can you do anything for neurogenic claudication?
23. How long does a cortisone shot take to wear off?

Treatment Modalities

1. Should I use ice or heat on my neck?
2. How does PIR (Post Isometric Relaxation) work?
3. What are the crackling sounds when you use that tool [Instrument assisted soft tissue]?
4. How long should I ice for?
5. Do you like ice or heat better?
6. Is IASTM good to use right before a lift?

7. For pin-and-stretch, is it better to move fast or slow?
8. Can electro-acupuncture help with muscle atrophy?
9. Is foam-rolling good for you?
10. What does kinesio-taping do?
11. What does electrical stimulation do?
12. Is there a reason why they put menthol in a lot of your lotions?
13. How do you feel about muscle tempering?
14. Should I be sore after practicing Bruegger's position?
15. Is my hip-popping sound a sign of instability?
16. What's the difference between traction and an inversion table?
17. How does flexion-and-distraction work?
18. Can you use a stim unit on genitals or would it hurt too much?
19. How does cupping work?
20. How does Acupuncture work?
21. How is dry-needling different from acupuncture?
22. Can cupping (and IASTM) help with cellulite and wrinkles?
23. *Patient with stenosis* Do I have to avoid all extension exercises?

Sleep

1. What's the best position to sleep in?
2. Is there a certain type of pillow that you recommend?
3. Should I use a soft or a hard mattress for my back?
4. Is there a good position for overweight people to sleep in?
5. Why am I SO thirsty when I wake up in the middle of the night?
6. What are some tips for sleeping better?
7. What's the best sleeping position for a pregnant patient?

Exercise

1. *Patient with a cold*-Would you recommend I work out today?
2. Does physical therapy work if you're not doing the exercises at home too?
3. Can I tear a muscle riding a bike?
4. Why does my low back feel stiff after a workout?
5. Are there any movements at the gym that I should avoid right now?
6. Can deadlifts cause disc herniations?
7. Are sit-ups dangerous?
8. Why do I get headaches after some workouts?

9. What rehab equipment should I buy for home?
10. What's anterior pelvic tilting?
11. What are some safe exercises and stretches for a pregnant patient?
12. Should I avoid holding my kid for now?

Random Things

1. Can a transgender woman have babies?
2. What chemicals are present when there's inflammation?
3. How do you feel about stem-cell therapy?
4. How do they test for cortisol levels?
5. Is my pain relief stunted because of acclimation to my morphine pump?
6. Why do I yawn when I'm out of breath?
7. Are you familiar with foot reflexology?
8. Why are dead bodies so limp?
9. How much sun exposure is too much?
10. Can the flu shot make your muscles sore?

3

Medical conditions

These are the conditions that the 1st 100 patients either had in the past or had when I saw them. I would recommend looking at these and thinking of what you would do for each of them (if applicable) or looking the condition up if you're not familiar with it!

Musculoskeletal

1. Sprains
    a. Ankle
    b. Wrist
    c. Cervical spine
    d. Lumbar spine
2. Strains
    a. Erector spinae
    b. Quadratus lumborum
    c. Trapezius
    d. Levator scapulae
    e. Latissimus dorsi
    f. Quadriceps
    g. Serratus anterior
    h. Anterior tibialis

3. Tears
    a. Achilles
    b. Latissimus dorsi
    c. Biceps
    d. Vastus lateralis
    e. AC joint
    f. ACL
    g. Meniscus
    h. Glenoid labrum
    i. Supraspinatus
    j. Wrist flexors
    k. UCL
4. Fractures
    a. Metatarsal
    b. Mandible
    c. Femur
    d. Clavicle
    e. Radius
    f. Tibia
    g. Fibula
    h. Spinous process (C5-C7)
    i. Skull
    j. Calcaneus (stress)
    k. Olecranon
5. Surgeries
    a. Discectomy
    b. Tommy John
    c. Pilonidal cyst removal
    d. Laboratomy

e. Eblation
f. Gum grafting
g. Terminal Ileum removal
h. Appendicitis / Appendectomy
i. Cholecystitis / Cholecystectomy
j. Vasectomy
k. Breast augmentation
l. Tonsillitis / Tonsillectomy
m. Fasciotomy
n. Septoplasty
o. Bowel obstruction
p. Lap band
q. Plate on clavicle
r. Spinal fusions
    i. Cervical
    ii. Lumbar
    iii. Lumbosacral
s. Arthroscopy
    i. Foot
    ii. Hand
    iii. Knee
    iv. Hip
    v. Shoulder
t. Replacements
    i. Knee
    ii. Hip

6. Tension Headaches / Migraines
7. Osteoporosis
8. Testicular torsion

9. Dislocations
    a. Posterior shoulder
10. Congenital Anomalies
    a. Double collar bone
11. Iliotibial Band Syndrome
12. DeQuervain's tenosynovitis
13. Negative Ulnar variance
14. Bone spurs
15. Bakers cyst
16. Pes Planus (flat foot)
17. Sciatica
18. Bursitis
    a. Trochanteric
    b. Shoulder
19. Scoliosis
20. Thoracic Outlet Syndrome
21. Frozen shoulder
22. Shoulder impingement
23. Compartment syndrome
24. Temporomandibular Disorder
25. Shoulder / Scapular dyskinesia
26. Osgood Schlatter's
27. Little leaguer's elbow
28. Deviated septum
29. Loose patella
30. Chondromalacia
31. Hernia
    a. Hiatal
    b. Femoral

c. Inguinal
d. Double
32. Cancer / tumors
a. Breast
b. Brain
c. Ear
d. Thyroid
e. Melanoma
f. Osteoid osteoma
33. Spinal stenosis
a. Cervical spine
b. Lumbar spine
34. Disc-Related
a. Bulges
i. Cervical
ii. Lumbar
b. Herniations
i. Cervical
ii. Lumbar
c. Degenerative disc disease
35. Neuropathy
36. Neurogenic claudication
37. Radiculopathy
a. Cervical spine
b. Lumbar spine
38. Arthritis
a. Cervical spine
b. Lumbar spine
c. Wrist

      d. Knee
39. Tendonitis/osis
      a. Biceps
      b. Achilles
      c. Trapezius
      d. Iliopsoas
      e. Plantar
      f. Wrist
40. Postural abnormality
41. Calcified hematoma
42. Rhabdomyolysis
43. Meralgia Paresthetica
44. Femoral Acetabular Impingement
45. Sinding-Larsen-Johansson disease

Non-Musculoskeletal

1. Obesity
2. Crohn's
3. Gynecomastia
4. CSF leakage
5. Mitral valve repair
6. Asthma
7. Concussion
8. Iron-deficiency anemia
9. Celiacs
10. Hashimoto's
11. Lyme's
12. Pregnant

13. Diabetes
    a. Type I
    b. Type II
14. Vitamin D deficiency
15. Medullary Sponge Kidney
16. Chicken pox, mumps, measles, shingles, mono
17. Eczema
18. Anxiety / Depression
19. Urinary Tract Infections
20. Thalassemia Minor
21. Hyperhomocysteinemia
22. Opioid addiction
23. Hypertension
24. Lymphedema
25. GERD
26. Viral meningitis
27. Splenomegaly
28. Hydronephrosis
29. Brain aneurysm
30. Gestational thrombocytopenia
31. Carotid stenosis
32. Bronchitis
33. Tonsillitis
34. Pregnancy complications
    a. Hemorrhaging during birthing
    b. C-sections
    c. Post-pregnancy Incompetent cervix
35. Medical implants

    a. Morphine pump
    b. Insulin pump
36. Shrapnel deposits
37. Advil-induced gastric ulcers
38. Polycystic Kidney Disease
39. Anorexia
40. Ventricular tachycardia
41. Gout
42. IgG Subclass II Deficiency
43. Eosinophilic Esophagitis (EoE)

4

Things We Didn't Know / Expect

The following is a list of things we did not expect. It's broken down into three different categories: patients, insurance, and business.

About Patients

1. Patients have lots of questions.
    a. As seen earlier, people will ask you lots of questions, especially about what you're doing with them and how it's helping them.
    b. People will also ask you advice on almost every other condition they have (musculoskeletal related or not) and see if there's anything you can do to help it.
2. Some patients will come very prepared
    a. Many patients will come in with a clear idea of the diagnosis they believe they have. They'll bring in print-outs of articles that support

their belief. They do their research and come in prepared.

3. Things are never cut-and-dry.
    a. Diagnoses can have conflicting symptoms. No one ever really appears with a "textbook" case, there's usually at least one curveball.
    b. Treatment that works for one person might not help another. Everyone's pain and condition is different, so although one technique or modality helped one person, it might not be as beneficial for someone with a very similar presentation.
4. There's confusion about Chiropractic.
    a. Initially, a lot of patients didn't really have a good idea of what chiropractic was or how it could benefit them. There's still the old-school stigma against it in that they think all we do is "crack" them.
    b. They loved to see that they went through a thorough initial exam and that there's way more to chiropractic than just adjustments (such as soft tissue work and rehabilitation) and that we can offer a lot for a wide variety of conditions.

About Insurance

1. How to join Insurance companies.
    a. The whole process of becoming credentialed with insurance companies was of course, entirely new to me. The first thing you have to do is fill out the CAQH (Council for Affordable Quality Healthcare). After that, you must fill out individual submission forms to the insurance companies you want to join. The companies will then look at your CAQH and determine if they will credential you or not.
    b. When joining individual insurance companies, I didn't know there are "umbrella" companies that encompass a wide variety of insurances. For instance, "Optum" encompasses United and Oxford. So instead of individually applying to them, you apply to Optum to get credentialed for all the ones that fall under that umbrella company.
2. How long it takes to join them.
    a. To become credentialed takes A LOT longer than I expected (25-90 days). Some are faster than others, but 3 months was the total time it took for

me to get fully credentialed with all the ones I applied to.

b. Don't plan on being paid from insurances for another 2-4 weeks after you become credentialed. I didn't get my first insurance check until week 16 of being open.

3. Some insurances require clinical submissions.

a. For some insurance companies, you need to submit a clinical note online before you can bill for a patient covered by them. Once you do that, they give you how many visits and for how long they will cover services (ex: "8 visits covered until 12/12/2017"). Without this clinical note, your services won't be covered. Make sure you know if that submission is needed before you bill the insurance company.

4. Some of the insurance terms are confusing.

a. There were a few terms and concepts that took some getting used to, such as figuring out copays (set cash amounts, like "$25/visit"), coinsurance (a percentage of what that plan covers, such as "20% of contract price"), and learning about different deductibles (there are in-network and out-of-network types). Most plans require the patient to pay the copay or co-insurance amount until the deductible has been met.

5. Some things on Electronic Health Records (EHR).
    a. I didn't know that the process of joining an EHR requires a lot of hands-on-practice (25 hours of training).
    b. There are free ones, but if you want to accept insurance you should get one that has all the best services, since they help you with your submissions and ANY questions you have. With that however, comes a price. Mine was an initial cost of $4,000 + $180/month.
6. What Clearing Houses were.
    a. I literally had no idea what a clearing house was. It's basically a company where you can submit all your insurance claims (from BCBS, United, Oxford, Cigna, etc.) to and they handle separating them and submitting them to the correct location. It saves a TON of stress and time. I ended up choosing Availity and I really like them.

b. Since I didn't know what it was, I also didn't know the expenses that come along with it, which is about $100/month.

About Business

1. Figuring out how many of everything to get.
    a. I had a pretty good idea of what equipment I wanted, but when it came time I realized I never went over how *much* of everything to get. I needed to know how many lotions to get, how many towels I needed, how many acupuncture needles to get, etc. And since we have a gym in our space, we needed to decide how many barbells, dumbbells, or medicine balls to buy. Drew and I decided to look at other offices and count and see how many of everything other people had and tailor that number to our situation.
    b. We created a shared google sheets document to continually update the equipment list and number. This then allowed us to see how fast we would go through things and how often we needed to re-order them.

2. Figuring out how to pay for everything.
   a. From there, I wasn't entirely sure how I was going to pay for it all. I ended up getting my equipment leased through Script Hesco and I have no complaints, they have great rates for new graduates.
3. There were unexpected expenses.
   a. There were many unexpected expenses that we didn't know about. For instance, for my EHR system we needed a strong enough computer, so we had to purchase one that could sustain it. There were also fees for starting an LLC and obtaining building permits, which we never really considered beforehand.
   b. We created our own projected expenses sheets with information obtained through various chiropractors and gym owners (i.e. cable, internet, insurance costs). This helped us more accurately forecast our projected operating expenses each month.
4. Some items are taxable.
   a. We didn't consider that some items, such as supplements or even personal

training are taxable. So, we had to choose whether to absorb and pay those taxes ourselves, or add the taxed price to the items.

5. The beginning phases of opening a new business.
    a. Working with landlord / zoning committees / getting approval
        i. There's a bunch of formal meetings and negotiations (such as lease negotiations) that take place before a letter of intent is solidified and the space is yours.
        ii. Then, there are certain codes that need to be followed, such as having a handicap accessible bathroom, having a certain amount of parking spots available for a medical office, and only using a certain amount of square footage for window signage based on the size of the space.
    b. Building out
        i. The process was a lot harder than expected. We had the help of an amazing contractor who walked us through it.

Between the 3 of us and an additional carpenter it took 2 months of working 10+ hours a day for 7 days/week before we were all set. Keep in mind that if you don't want to do any elbow work, you'll have to pay a premium. We saved tens of thousands by doing it ourselves.

c. Getting inspections

    i. Once you have your place and set it to code, you must pass certain inspections before you can open, including plumbing, electrical, and fire. From there, you will have to get a certification of occupancy that shows you passed all the inspections and you're finally ready to roll!

5

Recommendations

The following is a list of recommendations. Once again, they are broken down into three categories: patients, insurance, and business.

For Patients

1. Be patient-centered
   a. Try and understand the patient's perspective on the situation. A lot of them are truly scared. I've had patients tell me they were afraid they wouldn't be able to play with their kids or enjoy basic activities of their life because of the pain they experience. Listen carefully to their worries and fears and be empathetic towards them.
2. Have major referrals in line.
   a. *Know where you want to send them for imaging, blood work, referrals, etc.* There will be plenty of times where getting an image or sending out for a referral is necessary, and you don't

want to have to be scrambling around on where to send the patient.

    b. Also, *get familiar with the process of referring for an image*. Most of the imaging centers just require filling out an online form and then submitting it. From there the imaging center will contact and schedule the appointment with the patient.

3. Be prepared to treat.

    a. *Have an idea of what to do when a certain condition walks in*. For good practice, try creating a treatment plan for the conditions mentioned above. People REALLY appreciate when you can examine and start treating them (even just a little bit) on the same day. By having an idea of what to do for each condition, it becomes a lot easier and less stressful to do that.

4. Explain your treatment.

    a. Patients want to know what you're doing and why. By having a clear and simple explanation for your treatment, it puts them on the same page as you and allows them to understand what you're doing. It gives them a sense of comfort that is crucial in a visit to a doctor. *Do whatever you can to explain*, whether it be providing print-outs, having research articles available, drawing, etc.

5. Review each case before the visit.
    a. You want to be completely fresh on what's going on with each case. During the visit, you don't want to have to try to remember which side had the radiation and which didn't. *Re-read the last visit note and get yourself mentally-prepped.*
6. Know when to get an image.
    a. *Know when it's necessary to get an image.* Make sure you know the red flags, and go over extremity protocols as well. There was one month that was basically "ankle month," where I had a swarm of patients come in with swollen ankles. I had to review the Ottawa ankle rules a few times, but that's the beauty of Google.
7. Be familiar with the major different diets.
    a. People will ask you a lot of questions about all sorts of diets (Ketogenic, Paleo, Atkins, DASH, etc.), *so try and learn as much as you can about as many of them as possible.* You'll have patients come in that are on every diet you can think of.

8. Don't stop learning.
   a. When a patient comes in with a condition or past treatment that you're not familiar with, look it up, because chances are high that you'll see that again. For example, I couldn't remember what lithotripsy was, so I looked it up. The next day I had a new patient who recently had it done, so it allowed for an easy conversation about it.
   b. Like I mentioned in the "things I didn't expect" chapter, patients will ask you advice on almost every condition they or a relative have. *The more you learn the more you will be to help them.*
9. Take advantage of clinic time
   a. If you're still in school, learn as much as you can about each condition you encounter. You won't have as much time as you do there to study all you can. Devote some time to go in on other interesting cases that your classmates have. Learn from your clinicians and ask them as many questions as possible. Don't waste time on Facebook or YouTube, take advantage of your breaks and learn!

10. Focus on quality
    a. Do the best you possibly can for every patient. *Focus on quality first.* Quality leads to quantity.
11. Be yourself.
    a. *Don't try and be someone you're not.* If you're not familiar with a condition or treatment, just be honest with the patient. Tell them you'll look more into their case and will create the best treatment plan you can for them, even if it means referring them out.
12. Stay relaxed
    a. What will you say if a patient says, "I haven't been feeling any better, actually after last visit I've felt a little worse"? Be prepared to explain that your treatment might not be what that individual person needs. The fact of the matter is *not all patients will respond to care, but it's not necessarily your fault.*
13. Trust yourself
    a. It's normal to feel overwhelmed and "not ready yet," but you know more than you think you know. Focus on applying all the things you've learned in an easily explainable manner. *There's going to be a learning curve,*

but understand that, trust the process, and trust yourself.

14. Be patient

    a. You can't be a doctor without any patience (pun intended). A big thing I've learned this past year is that I needed to wait until I established a significant base (for me of about 85 people) until there was a large amount of word-of-mouth referral of new patients every moth. Until then, you want to have a strong focus on efforts that offer immediate return (fast new patients). Now location and signage are very important for this, since they offer 24/7 coverage for you, but outside of that there are plenty of other options. Personally, I focused on treating "influencers" – people who can refer a large number of patients (such as other docs in different fields, head personal trainers, gym owners, business owners, etc.). The goal should be to get to that large patient base as fast as possible, and I found that 3-5 good influencers can easily add 3-6 new patients each. For example, when I first opened, my sister (who has a couple thousand followers on Instagram) made a short "Instagram story" showing me working on her. Within the next 2 days I had 3 new patients come in just from seeing that. While most of your focus is on that immediate return, I recommend maintaining a small, but consistent effort on more long-term returns – such as blogs, social media posts, etc. Until I got that patient base, these things only drew a small number of patients. But once that base is large enough, you want to make sure you have a good amount of material for them and others (all while building your brand). *Be focused on building that base, but be patient and know that when you get there it gets much easier.*

For Insurance

1. Get your NPI number
   a. Your NPI (National Provider Identification) number is required once you start practicing. It's really easy to get online and *should be completed as soon as possible.*

2. Fill out the CAQH immediately
    a. The CAQH is a giant online resume that is required if you want to join insurance companies, or if you're joining a practice that accepts insurance. The CAQH acts like a "common application" for insurance companies to look at and decide if they want to accept you as an in-network provider.
3. Know which insurance companies you want to join
    a. Know what each company pays, what they require, etc. Some offer per-visit compensation ($60/visit) while others offer per-service ($35 for an adjustment, $20 for manual therapy, etc.). *Know what to expect and which ones you want to be a part of.*
4. Know which EHR and clearing house you want to use.
    a. *Figure out which EHR you want and start the required training / practicing as soon as you can.* You want to get comfortable with it as soon as possible so you don't have to spend time doing that instead of focusing on patients. I ended up choosing 1st

Provider's Choice and I love them. The staff is extremely helpful and allows you to develop a strong and familiar relationship with them.

5. Know how to check patient benefits
   a. This is a big one. When someone walks in, how will you know what their benefits are - did they hit their deductible, how many visits do they get, etc.? You can call the insurance company (which is very time-consuming for each patient), but I recommend checking if your EHR or clearing house has an online service where you can check the benefits out immediately.

For Business

1. Be as prepared as possible.
   a. This is the most important thing if you plan on opening. "Victory favors neither the righteous nor the wicked; only the prepared." *Have a well-thought-out business plan that includes EVERYTHING* (marketing plans, mission statement, demographics, competition, expected expenses, services provided, profits and losses, prices, etc.) and draw out

your blueprint based on the square footage you have. If you're trying to raise money in any way (loan or investment), *everyone* will ask to see the business plan. Having a thorough and in-depth one will only benefit you. We spent countless hours working on ours and it helped once people realized how much thought we put into it.

2. Start small.
   a. We originally planned on opening a 3,000-sq. ft. facility, but luckily one of our mentors asked us why we couldn't start our business in a smaller space. We listened to his advice and started with an 1100-sq. ft. space and it has been tremendously helpful. The overhead cost is way cheaper than it would have been, and we haven't had any trouble utilizing the smaller space. *It's much better to be able to expand rather than be forced to downsize.*

3. Location is everything.
   a. This couldn't be truer. Having a prime location sets the stage for an increased number of potential patients. *Make sure your place is easily visible and accessible,* has

plenty of parking available, and is placed in an area that is surrounded by similar businesses. We lucked out with our location. We're right in the heart of an up-and-coming area, underneath an apartment complex, and adjacent to a major aquarium, yoga studio, and juice bar.

4. Get systems in check.
    a. What social media outlets will you use? *Set up social media accounts and come up with a social media marketing strategy.* If you can develop the habit of thinking about and posting on social media early on it will make life much easier once you get busy.
    b. How will you keep track of profits and losses? Our accountant helped us set up a QuickBooks account and it made life way easier for evaluating our company appropriately. *Try to have the basic systems of your company established.*

5. Have money saved.
    a. As mentioned earlier, there's going to be unexpected expenses, even in your personal life. For instance, my car took its last breath 4 months into

opening (R.I.P.), and I had to get a new one. Plan for that, and *have extra money saved.*

6. Have mentors.
    a. We wouldn't have been able to do anything if we didn't have the help of people who are familiar with running successful businesses. They know the ins-and-outs and can offer priceless advice and guidance. *Try to connect with 3-5 people* who you look up to and who are able to help you out with any questions you have.
7. Don't go too cheap.
    a. With everything you buy, *get good quality and don't go cheap*. Whether it be with toilet paper, cleaning wipes, whatever. People judge the small things and they WILL notice. Keep the office as clean as possible and keep it neat and professional. Keeping the place clean can be annoying and tedious, but it's well worth it.
8. Get a good logo.
    a. A nice logo can help shape the brand you want. It's an underrated aspect of your business and can help allow for easy recognition. We had a graphic designer create ours, and it was well

worth the price. *Put effort into creating your logo.*

9. Get great signage.
    a. Your signage is the one marketing tool that for a one-time price offers 24/7 coverage for potential patients. The week we got ours up there was a huge influx of people walking / calling in. *Make sure it clearly states who you are, what you do, and how to contact you.*
10. If you're building out, have a contractor help.
    a. *Try and find a contractor that you really trust and have him/her help you with building out the place.* They understand the process that goes along with it and can be instrumental in helping you.
11. Absorb necessary expenses.
    a. Opening a business requires a tight budget, but don't ignore expenses that can make or break you. Hiring people like an accountant or lawyer may seem like a pricey expense at first, but they can help you save lots of money in the long run. Our accountant has been by far one of our biggest assets.

12. Keep any business-class notes from school.
    a. At National University of Health Sciences, I had an excellent business professor and the amount of excellent information he provided was invaluable. That's how Drew and I got the business plan and profits-and-losses format started, from the class. Keep whatever information you think might be beneficial in the future.
13. Be relationship-oriented.
    a. Set your focus on developing strong relationships with people. Don't over-concern yourself with just trying to get as many people as possible in the door at the expense of delivering your full and highest quality of care.
14. Walk the walk.
    a. You're a walking billboard of your product. Patients really will trust you more if you follow your own advice.

About the Authors

Dr. Brandon Buchla DC, CSCS

Dr. Buchla graduated from Fordham University with a Bachelor's in Biology. He then received his Chiropractic degree from National University of Health Sciences. While there, he completed a 100-hour sports acupuncture and dry needling course through the Midwest Rehabilitation Institute and received his CSCS through the National Strength and Conditioning Association. After graduating in December 2016, he opened "A Team Performance and Chiropractic" with Drew 3 months later.

Drew Accomando CPT, FRC

Drew Accomando comes from a lifetime of health and fitness. Drew earned his degree in Health and Physical Education Teaching, while being a four-year varsity baseball letter-winner at Eastern Connecticut State University. As a two-year team captain team, Drew was also a four-year All-Little East Conference Academic Team member. A great amount of Drew's skill comes in sport performance, weight loss / transformation, special needs, and corporate / executive group training.

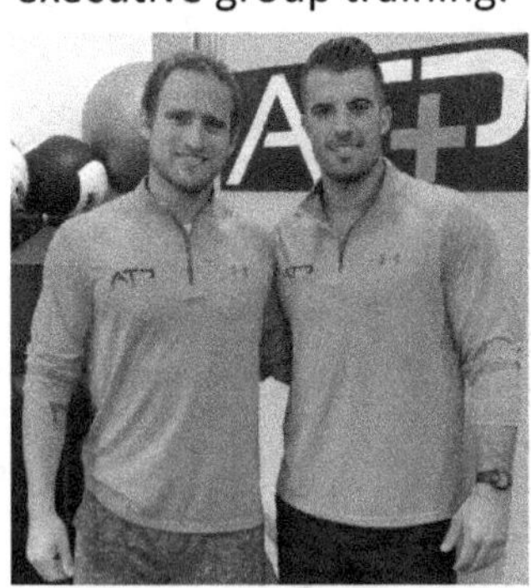

The ATP+ Story

ATP+ (A Team Performance and Chiropractic) has been a long-term goal for us. Drew and I became best friends in high school where we were on the football team together. We started working out outside of the scheduled hours and started to bond over our similar thoughts on training and sports. We decided early on that we would want to be working with each other. After we graduated college, Drew went on to become the head YMCA personal trainer while I went to and finished chiropractic school. Throughout those years, we kept working on and solidifying our business plan, and the second I graduated we already had a place in mind that we wanted. We signed the lease 3 weeks later and then got to work! This has been our dream for a long time, and we're unbelievably happy to watch it unfold.

Check us out!

Instagram: @atp.chiro
Website: www.atpplusct.com
Facebook: A Team Performance and Chiropractic

Cover and Back photo by Jackie Ryan (@jeryanx)

The First Year in Practice is a compilation of all the questions and conditions that the first 100 patients had after a 2016 graduate opened a private practice. It includes:

- >100 questions that were asked
- > 100 conditions that walked in
- A list of unexpected things and recommendations pertaining to patients, insurance, and business